Manual of hematology

Paul Richard Reich, M.D.
Assistant Professor of Medicine
Beth Israel Hospital
Harvard Medical School
Boston, Massachusetts

Sixth Edition
Reprinted 1978
Reprinted 1980
Reprinted 1982
Reprinted 1983
Reprinted 1985
Reprinted 1987
Published by The Upjohn Company

Upjohn

Contents

Myeloid Cells
Figures 1-8

Figure 1 Myeloblast
The myeloblast, the earliest white cell precursor, is characterized by scant cytoplasm, one or more nucleoli, and the absence of visible black or purple promyelocytic granules. Its diameter is 15-20 microns and the nucleus is round or oval. These cells are extremely difficult to differentiate from lymphoblasts.

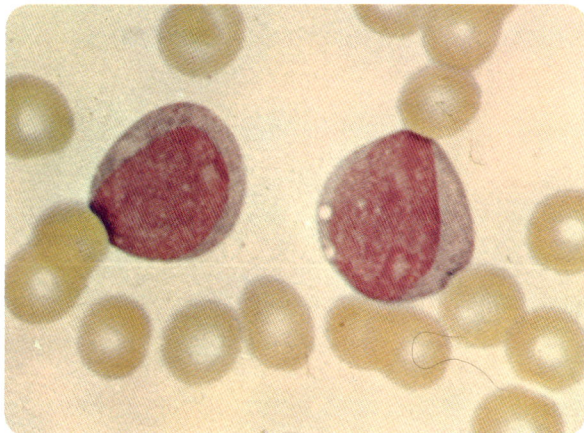

Figure 2 Promyelocyte
This cell is similar in appearance to the myeloblast. However, its cytoplasm contains large black or purple granules. Nucleoli may be present.

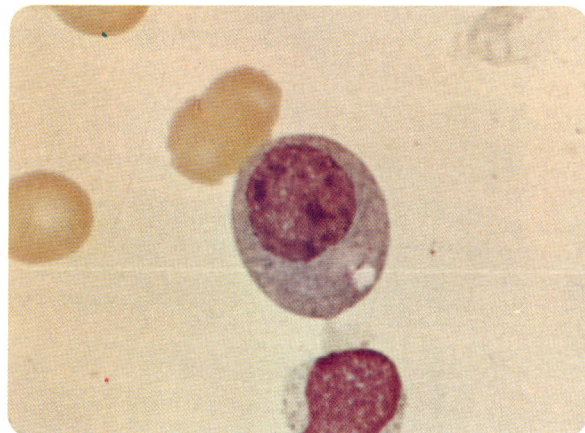

Figure 3 Myelocyte
Unlike the myeloblast and promyelocyte, the myelocyte's cytoplasm contains neutrophilic granules. The nucleus still has a round or oval shape, and no nucleoli are present. The large promyelocytic granules are not seen.

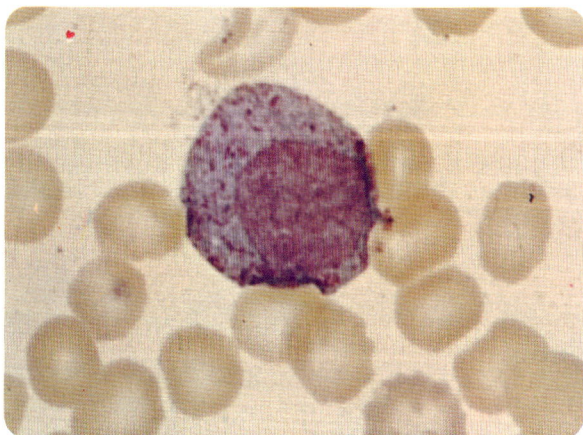

Figure 4 Metamyelocyte (juvenile)
This cell has a kidney-shaped nucleus; the cytoplasm contains neutrophilic granules and lacks promyelocytic granules.

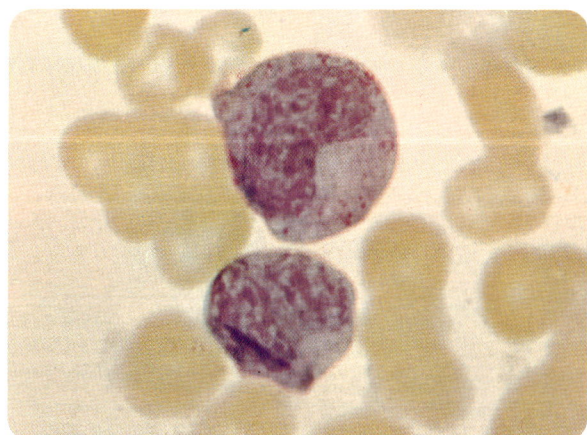

Figure 7   Basophil
The basophil on the right (neutrophil on the left) has cytoplasm and a nucleus similar to that of the mature leukocyte. However, the cytoplasm is filled with large, dark-purplish granules which may cover the cell's nucleus.

Figure 5   Band form (stab)
This myeloid element is similar to the metamyelocyte but the band form has a horseshoe-shaped nucleus.

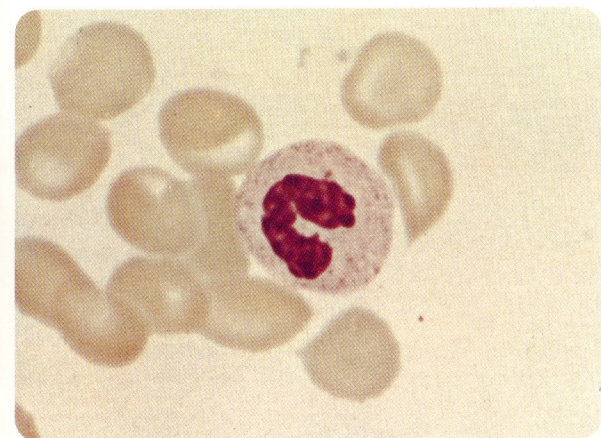

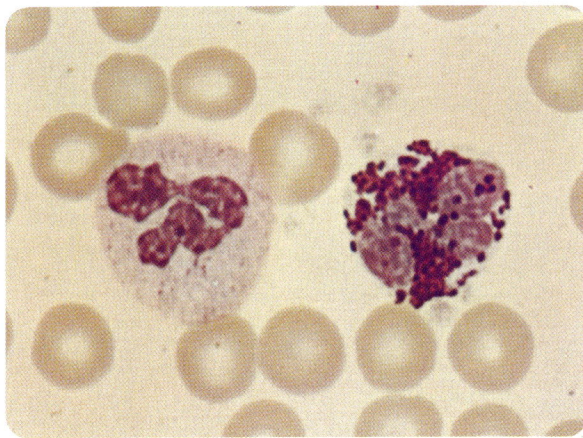

Figure 6   Segmented neutrophil (poly)
This cell is approximately 12 to 14 microns in diameter. The nucleus is lobulated, having two to five lobes connected by thin strands of chromatin.

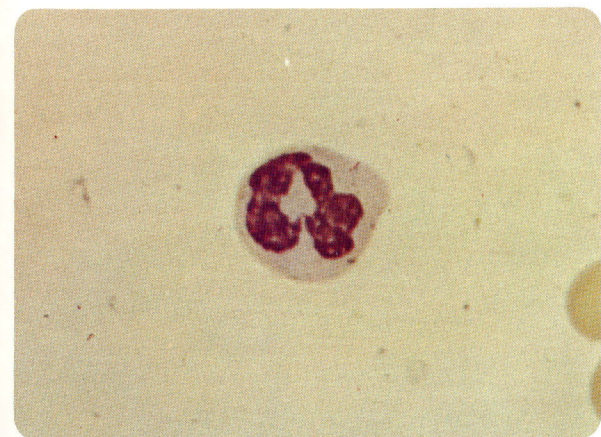

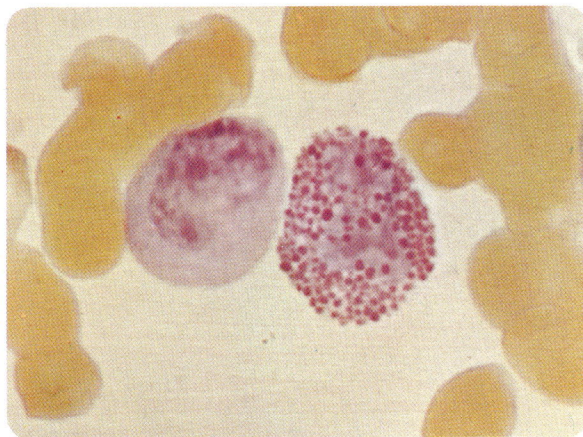

Figure 8   Eosinophil
This cell is characterized by the presence of numerous large, light-red granules which fill the cytoplasm and sometimes cover the nucleus. It is otherwise similar to the mature neutrophil.

Lymphocyte, Monocyte, and Plasma Cell

Figures 9-11

Figure 9   Lymphocyte

The lymphocyte has a "pale" blue cytoplasm and a dense, dark-staining nucleus. Depending on the amount of cytoplasm, the cell is classified as a large or small lymphocyte.

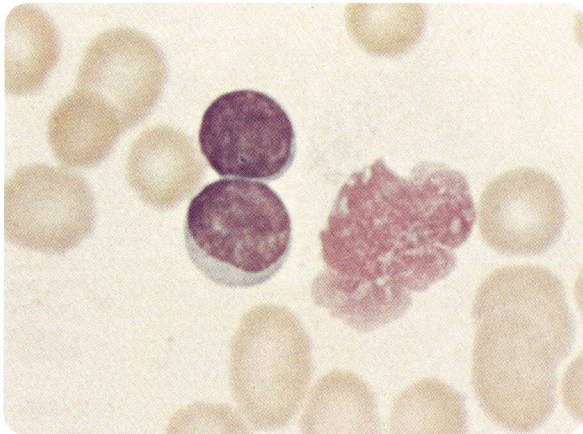

Figure 11   Plasma cell

A plasma cell is characterized by an eccentric nucleus, perinuclear clear zone, or pale-staining area adjacent to the nucleus and dark-purple cytoplasm.

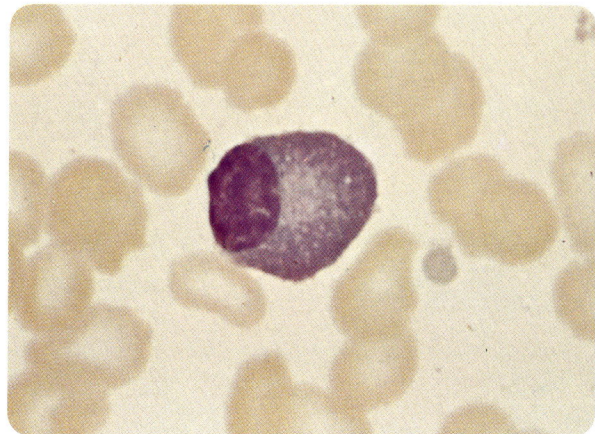

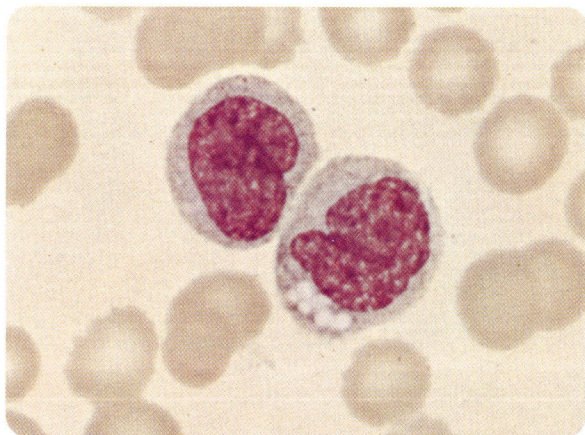

Figure 10   Monocyte

This cell has a blue-gray granular cytoplasm and a lobulated nucleus. It is distinguished from other leukocytes by the folding over of the nuclear lobes.

Erythroid Cells
Figures 12-16

Figure 12   Erythroblast (pronormoblast) *(right)*
This earliest erythroid precursor is a large cell (12-20 microns) with blue cytoplasm. It contains a finely reticular and multi-nucleolated nucleus. The reticular, mesh-like nucleus and dark-blue cytoplasm usually allow differentiation of erythroblasts from myeloblasts and lymphoblasts. The nuclear characteristics also distinguish it from a plasma cell.

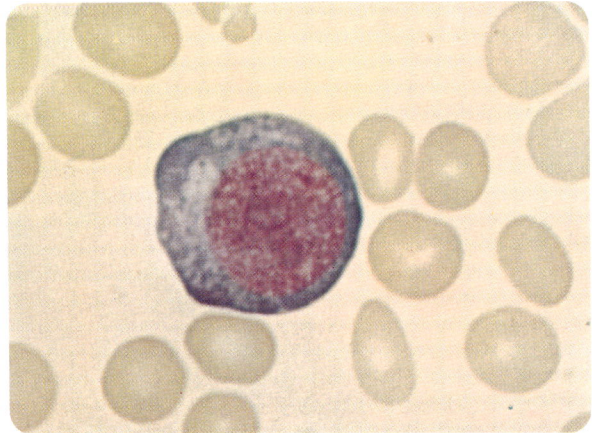

Figure 13   Basophilic normoblast *(below)*
This cell retains the blue cytoplasm seen in the erythroblast but nucleoli are not present and the nuclear chromatin is more clumped and densely stained. As maturation continues, the size of the erythroid precursor decreases from approximately 15 microns to about 10 microns.

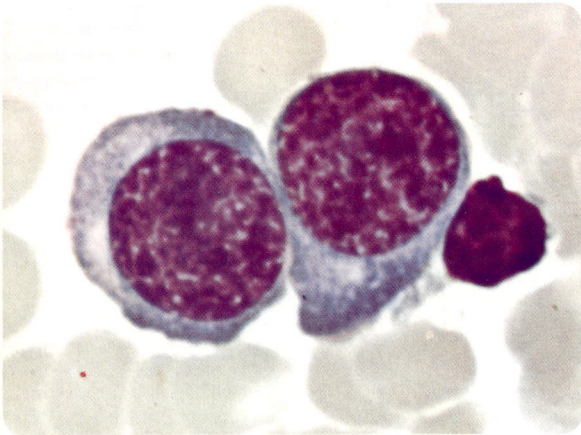

Figure 15   Orthochromatic normoblast *(below)*
A "nucleated red blood cell" with a pink or gray cytoplasm and a small pyknotic nucleus. Nucleated red cells are abnormal in peripheral blood, but may be present in patients with hemolytic anemia, leukemia, myeloproliferative syndrome, myelophthisic anemia, megaloblastic anemia and other severe anemias.

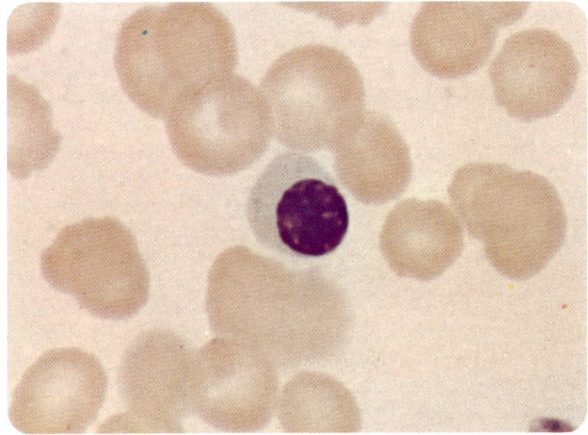

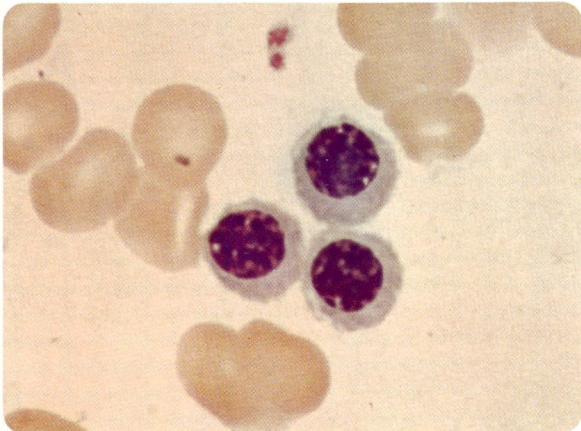

Figure 14   Polychromatic normoblast
The presence of hemoglobin is first seen in the polychromatic normoblast as pink material mixed with the cytoplasm. Its nucleus is smaller than that in the basophilic normoblast, with even more clumped chromatin.

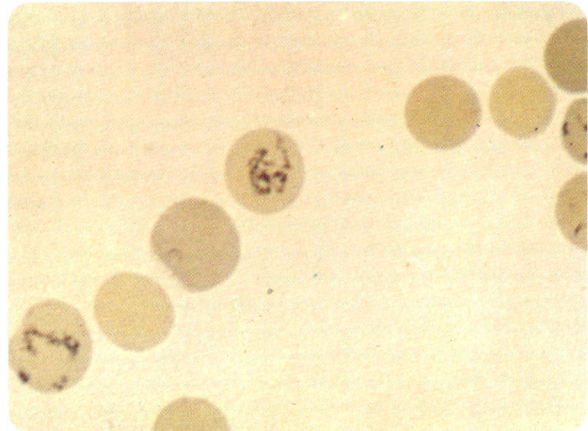

Figure 16   Reticulocytes
Newly formed erythrocytes, when stained supervitally with new methylene blue, contain a blue reticular (RNA) network. These cells appear as macrocytes with diffuse cytoplasmic basophilia (polychromasia) when stained with Wright stain.

Non-erythroid, Non-myeloid Cells
Figures 17-21

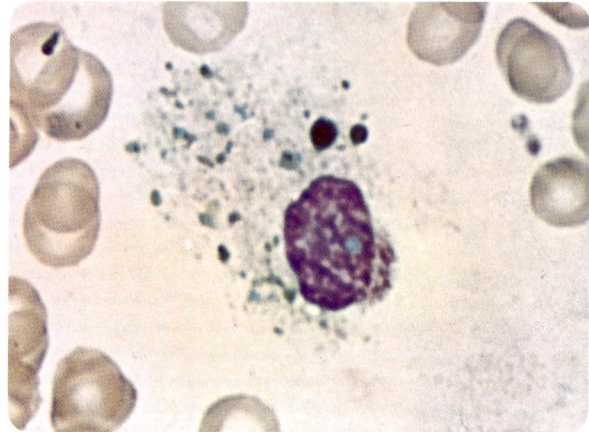

Figure 17   Reticuloendothelial cell *(right)*
This large cell (20-30 micron diameter) has a filmy cytoplasm, sometimes containing inclusions, and a nucleus with one or more bluish-colored nucleoli. Increased numbers are seen in marrows from patients with infectious, inflammatory, or malignant diseases.

Figure 18   Mast cell
Large, dense, black granules which completely fill the cytoplasm characterize this cell. These cells are found in increased numbers in the bone marrows of patients with osteoporosis and systemic mastocytosis.

Figure 20   Megakaryocyte *(below)*
This very large cell, with a multilobulated nucleus, is the progenitor of circulating platelets. The latter are usually seen streaming off the megakaryocyte's cytoplasm.

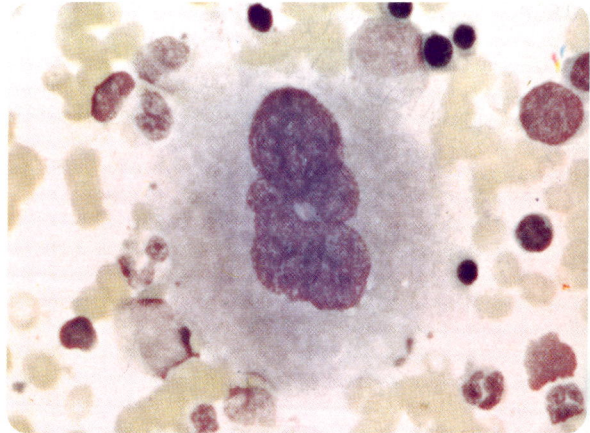

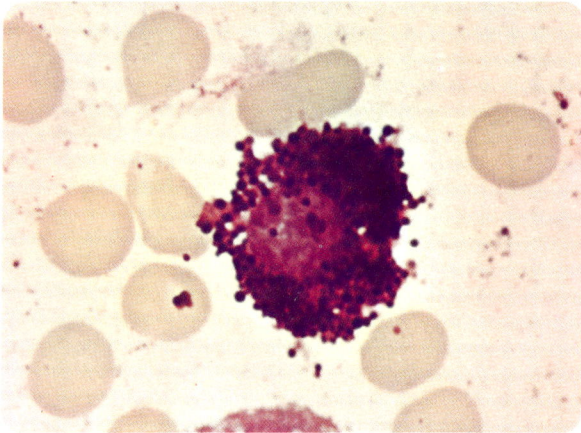

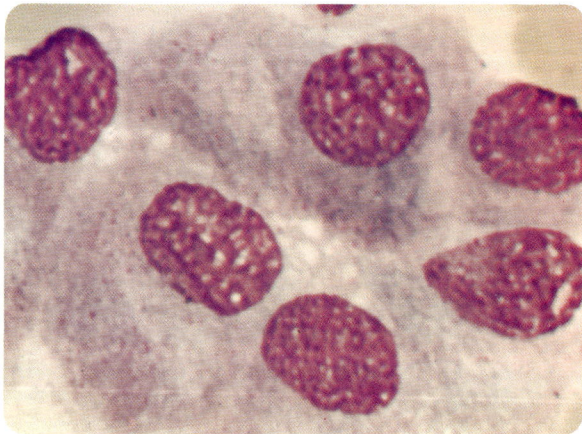

Figure 19   Osteoblast
These cells resemble plasma cells but their clear cytoplasmic area is distal from the nucleus, rather than perinuclear. They often appear in clumps and have been mistaken for tumor cells.

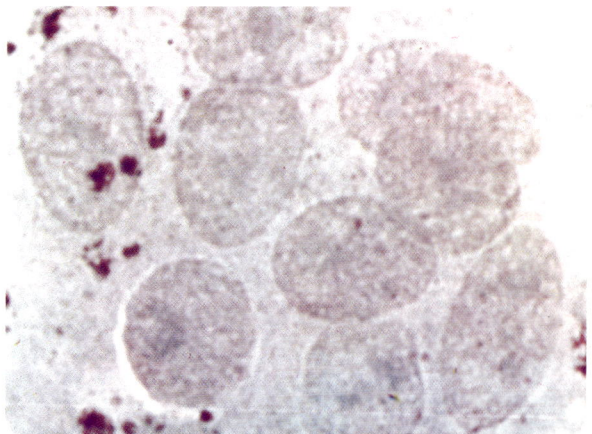

Figure 21   Osteoclast
This is a very large cell which is sometimes mistaken for a tumor cell. However, unlike a tumor cell, this cell has numerous nuclei, each of which contains nucleoli. They are more commonly seen in patients of the pediatric age group.

Myeloid Abnormalities
Figures 22 and 23

Figure 22   L.E. cell
The presence of a homogenous pink or purple nuclear material occupying the cytoplasm of a mature neutrophil, and displacing its nucleus to the periphery, is characteristic of the cell seen in systemic lupus erythematosus and other "collagen" diseases. Special procedures which traumatize leukocytes are used to demonstrate the cells in the buffy coat of blood from patients with these diseases.

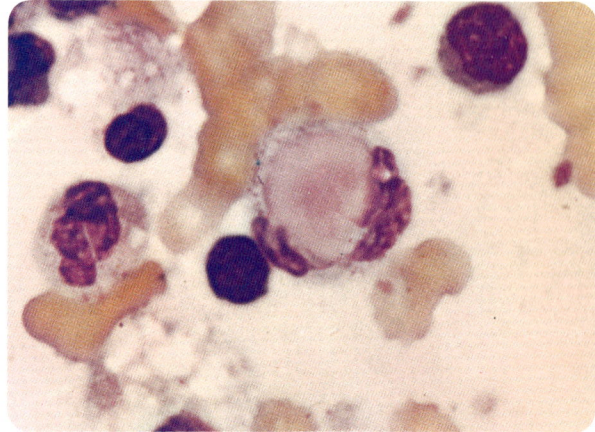

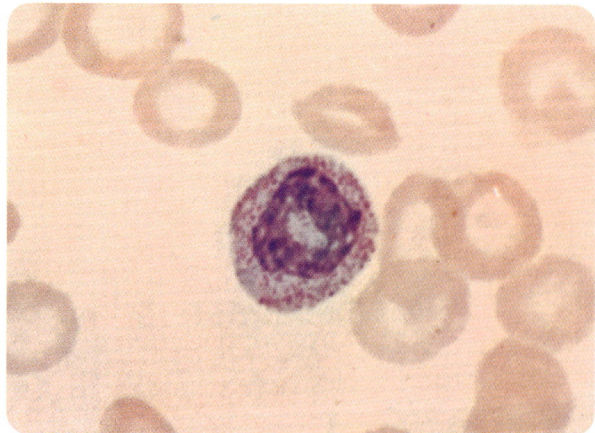

Figure 23   Toxic granulation and Döhle body
Patients ill with bacterial or viral infections often have dark-purple or black granules in the mature neutrophils. Also, blue RNA-containing inclusions, called Döhle bodies, appear in the cytoplasm, as seen at "seven o'clock" in this cell.

Myeloproliferative Diseases

Figures 24-31

Figure 24 Acute myelocytic leukemia

This disease is characterized by the presence of large numbers of myeloblasts in the peripheral blood and a large percentage of myeloblasts and promyelocytes in the bone marrow. The myeloblast is distinguished from the lymphoblast by the presence of Auer rods (Figure 25) or by mature granulocytic elements in association with the myeloblast. Myeloblasts may also be seen in the myeloproliferative syndrome and in leukemoid reactions.

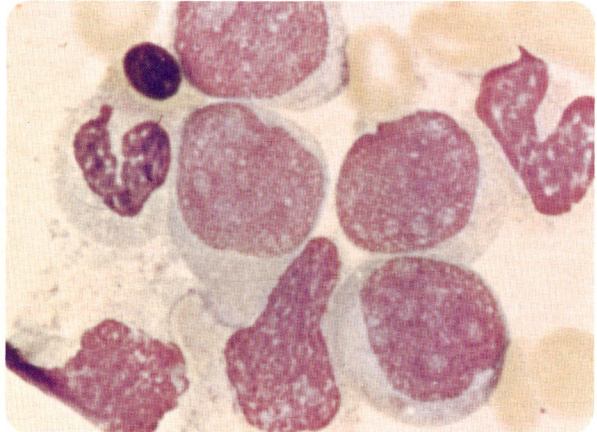

Figure 26 Acute monocytic leukemia

This leukemia is characterized by the presence of large numbers of cells having nuclear characteristics similar to those of monocytes; that is, the nucleus is lobulated and folded over on itself. The immaturity of these cells is suggested by the prominent nucleoli.

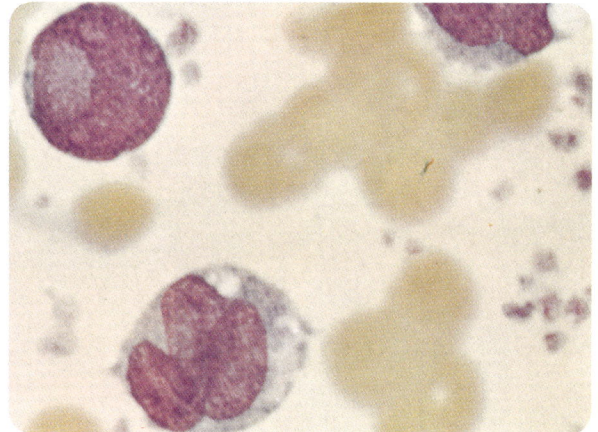

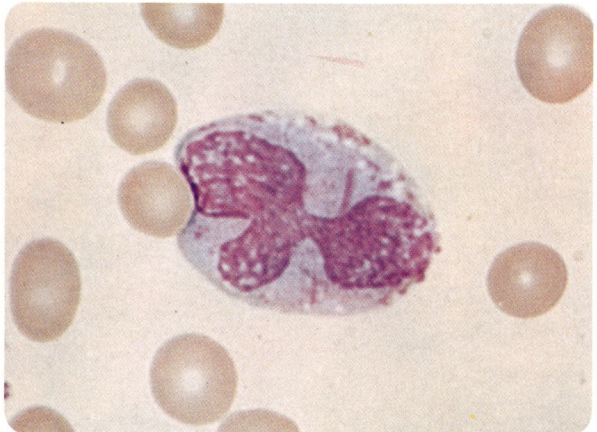

Figure 25 Auer rods

These cytoplasmic inclusions are round or rod-like in shape, one to six microns long, and have a red-purple color. They may be seen in acute myelocytic or myelomonocytic leukemia.

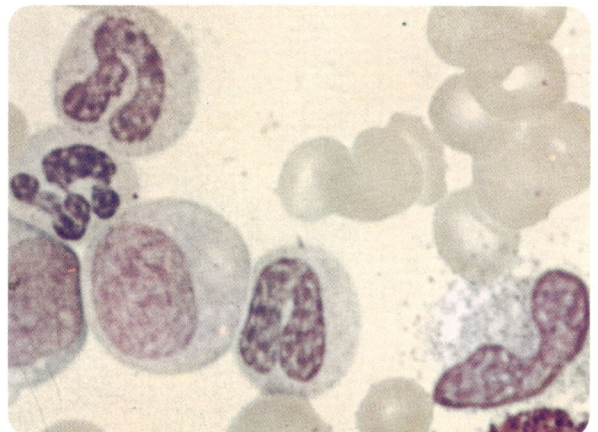

Figure 27 Chronic myelocytic leukemia

The peripheral blood is characterized by the presence of immature white blood cells including myeloblasts, promyelocytes, myelocytes, and metamyelocytes. Basophils are often increased in number. Erythroid precursors may also be seen.

Figures 28, 29, 30, 31 Myeloproliferative syndrome

The term "myeloproliferative syndrome" covers a group of diseases that are characterized by the presence of immature white cells in the peripheral blood and by erythroid abnormalities such as teardrop-shaped and nucleated red cells. The presence of immature white cells and nucleated red cells in the peripheral blood is sometimes referred to as a "leukoerythroblastic anemia." In the bone marrow, infiltration by fibroblasts and the presence of fibrosis is characteristic. Chronic myelocytic leukemia and agnogenic myeloid metaplasia often show at least some of these red and white cell abnormalities.

Figure 28
Immature white cells in the peripheral blood.

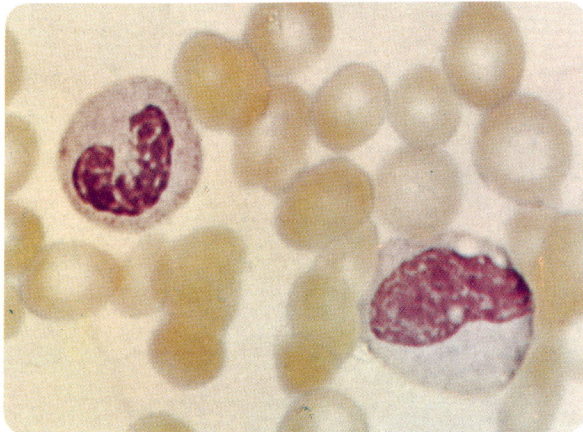

Figure 30
Teardrop cells in the peripheral blood.

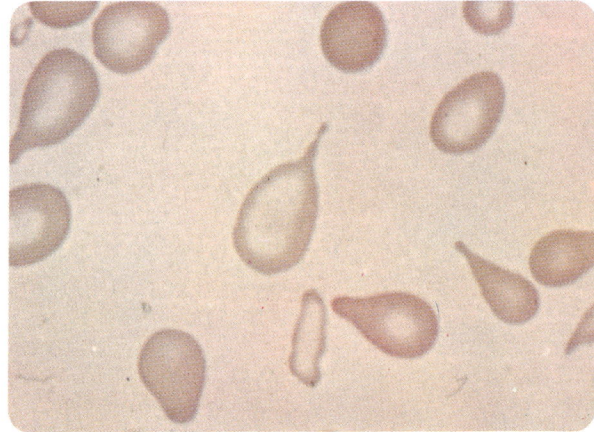

Figure 29 (x 675)
A bone marrow clot. Fibrotic material, stained blue with Masson's trichrome, has infiltrated the normal cellular elements.

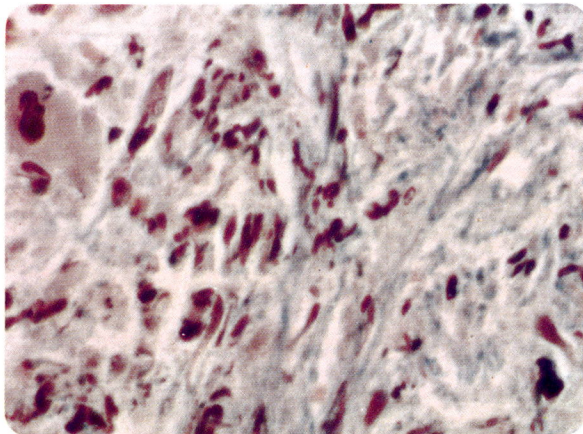

Figure 31
Nucleated red cell with "stippling" in the cytoplasm. Stippling of red cell cytoplasm may also be seen in hemolytic anemias, lead poisoning, and thalassemia as well as in the myeloproliferative syndrome.

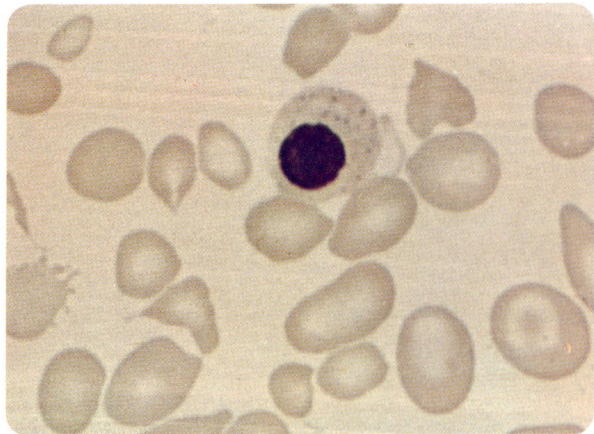

Lymphoproliferative Diseases

Figures 32-37

Figures 32, 33, 34 Infectious mononucleosis
The peripheral blood picture in this disease is characterized by the presence of large numbers of atypical lymphocytes. These lymphocytes are atypical in that they have vacuolated cytoplasm, nuclei which are folded over or lobulated like a monocyte, or their nuclei may contain nucleoli.

Figure 32
Atypical lymphocyte with many vacuoles in the cytoplasm.

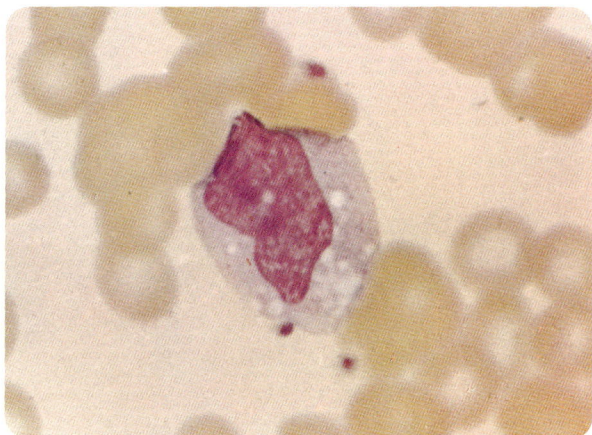

Figure 33
Atypical lymphocyte whose nucleus resembles that seen in a monocyte.

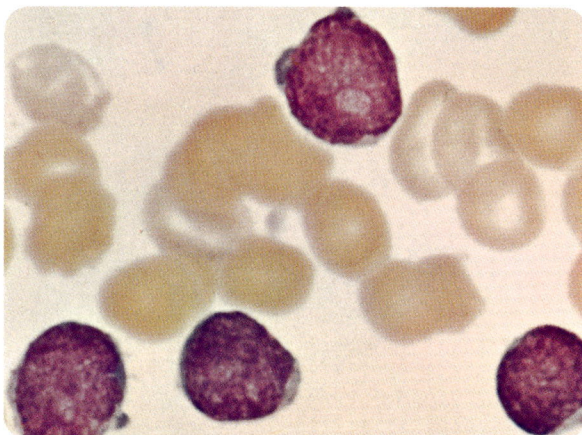

Figure 34
A distinct nucleolus is seen in this atypical lymphocyte's nucleus.

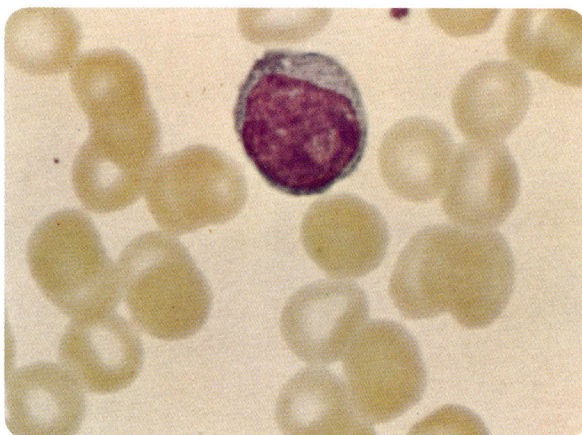

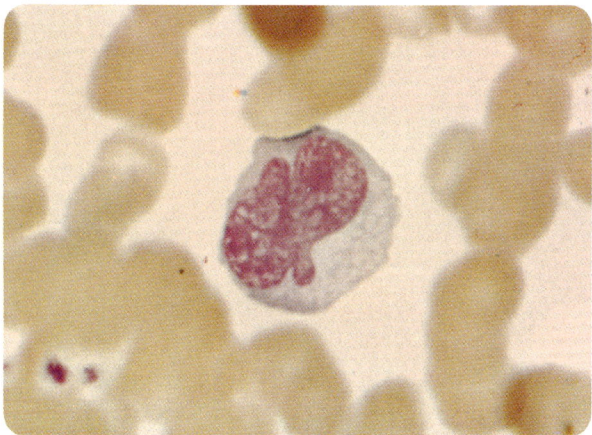

Figure 35 Acute lymphatic leukemia
The presence of lymphocytes and lymphoblasts (immature lymphocytes with nucleoli) characterizes the peripheral blood and bone marrow of patients with acute lymphatic leukemia. The cells are similar to those seen in chronic lymphosarcoma, cell leukemia, or chronic lymphatic leukemia. Acute lymphatic leukemia is generally found in children.

Figure 36   Chronic lymphatic leukemia
This disease of adults is characterized by the presence of large numbers of mature lymphocytes. Up to 5% of the cells may have nucleoli and resemble those seen in acute lymphatic leukemia or chronic lymphosarcoma cell leukemia. Smudge cells, which are clumps of eosinophilic material with an irregular outline, are often seen interspersed among the lymphocytes.

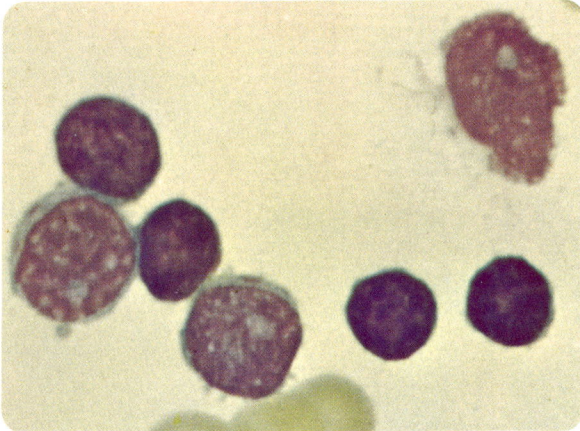

Figure 38   Multiple myeloma
Infiltration of the bone marrow by normal and immature plasma cells is characteristic of this disease. The atypical plasma cells are characterized by the presence of nucleoli in their nuclei and are called plasmablasts. Even more immature forms take on some of the characteristics of the reticuloendothelial cell. Various proportions of mature and immature cells are seen in the bone marrows of patients with this disease.

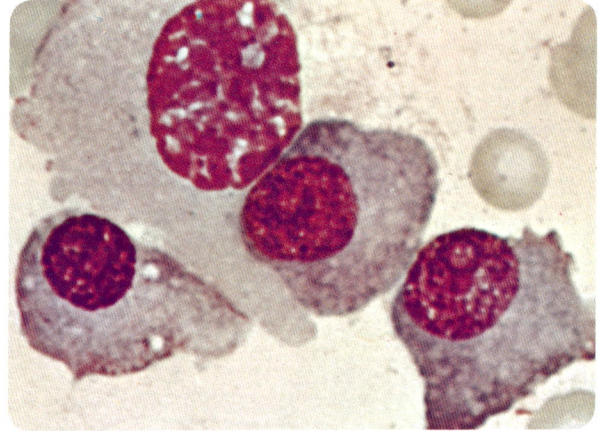

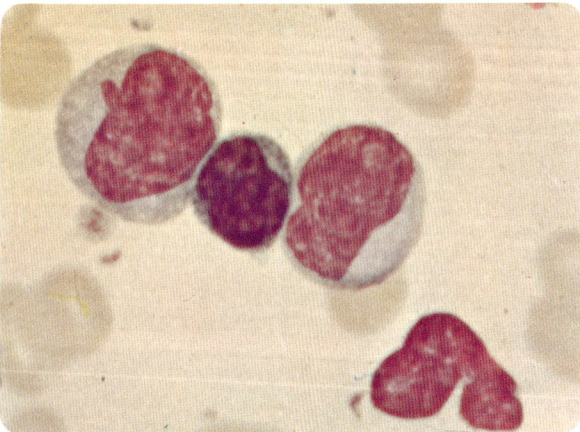

Figure 37   Chronic lymphosarcoma cell leukemia
In this subvariety of chronic lymphatic leukemia, more than 5% of the lymphocytes have a very atypical appearance. The nuclei are lobulated, folded over, clefted, or contain nucleoli. This disease generally carries a more unfavorable prognosis than chronic lymphatic leukemia.

Figure 39 Malignant lymphoma

Although malignant lymphoma is generally thought to be a disease of the lymph node, in many cases it involves the bone marrow. The characteristic appearance of this involvement, as seen on Wright-stained smears of bone marrow aspirates, is the presence of clumps of lymphocytes, lymphoblasts, and reticulum cells. A definite diagnosis usually requires lymph node or bone marrow biopsy.

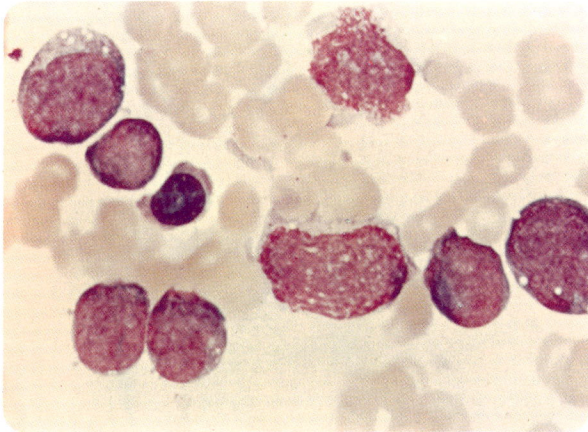

Figure 40 Macroglobulinemia

This disease is closely related to lymphoma and multiple myeloma. In this disease, abnormal macroglobulins are produced in large quantities. The typical cells seen in the bone marrow of these patients have features characteristic of both the plasma cell and lymphocyte. Nucleoli may be present. These cells are sometimes referred to as "plymphocytes."

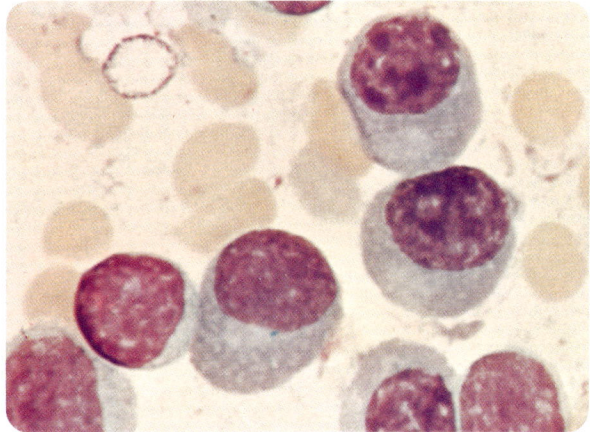

Figure 41 Gaucher's disease

This lipid storage disease is characterized by the presence of abnormal reticuloendothelial cells. These reticuloendothelial cells are filled with glucocerebroside which gives the cytoplasm a characteristic pale, foamy, or fibular appearance.

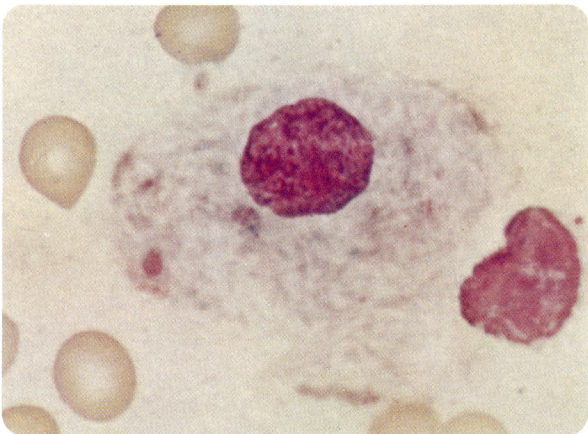

Figure 42 Tumor cells

Infiltration of the marrow by carcinoma is indicated by the presence of clumps of large cells with scant blue cytoplasm and nucleolated nuclei.

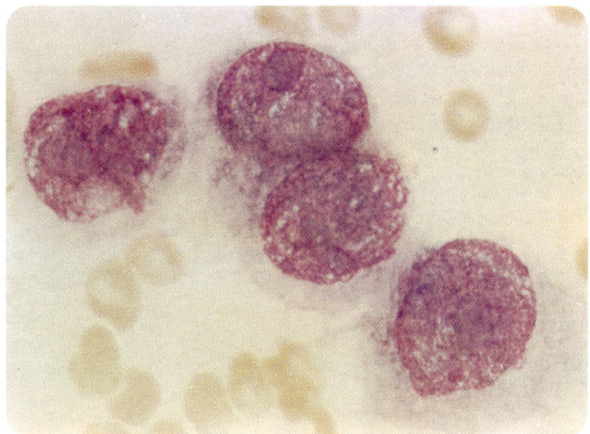

Diseases of Erythroid Cells
Figures 43-60

Figure 43   Hypochromic microcytic anemia

Small, pale cells, less than six microns in diameter, characterize this anemia. The pallor is due to a decreased concentration of hemoglobin. These cells are characteristically seen in iron deficiency anemia but may be present in the iron-loading anemias, the anemia of chronic disease, thalassemia, and lead poisoning.

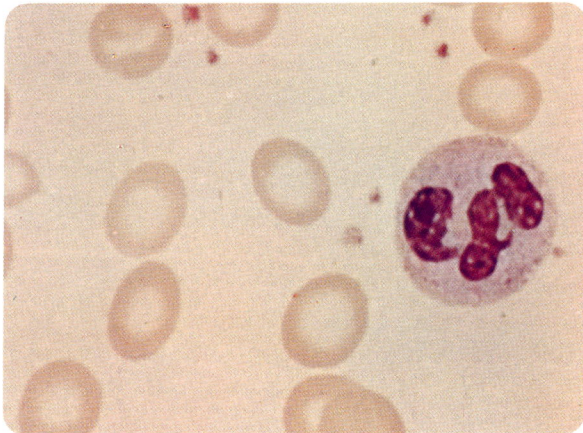

Figure 45   Megaloblastic anemia

These anemias are characterized by the presence of neutrophils with more than five nuclear lobes. Also characteristic is the presence of the large (greater than 8 microns in diameter), oval cells called macroovalocytes. Megaloblastic anemias are usually due to cyanocobalamin (B_{12}) or folic acid deficiency but characteristics of this anemia are also seen in red cells from patients with leukemia. Large round, not oval, cells called macrocytes may be seen in liver disease, hypothyroidism, hyperthyroidism, multiple myeloma, and in the normal newborn.

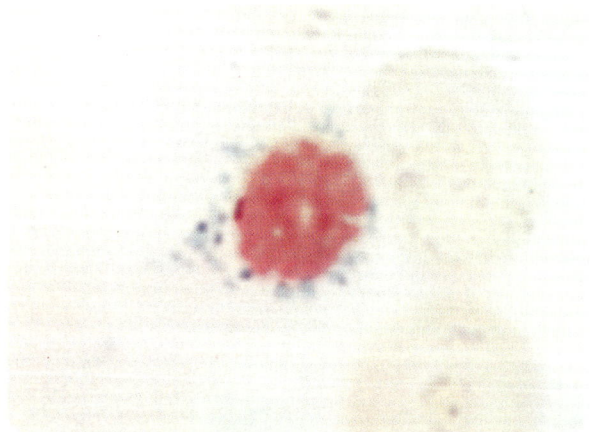

Figure 44   Ringed sideroblast

This cell is recognized in the bone marrow only after staining with Prussian blue for iron. They are normoblasts with a ring of blue mitochondrial iron arranged around the nucleus like a necklace. Bone marrows from patients with iron loading anemias, such as lead poisoning or sideroblastic anemias, thalassemia, megaloblastic anemia, leukemia, alcoholism, and following treatment with certain drugs may contain these cells.

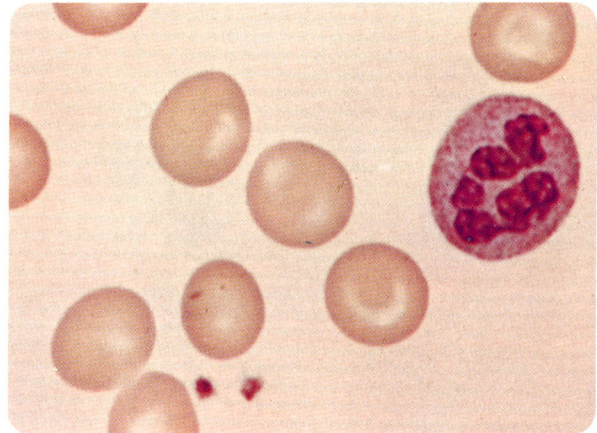

Figure 46   Megaloblast

This erythroid precursor is characterized by asynchrony between the young-appearing nucleus and the mature cytoplasm of the cell. Also characteristic is the stippled or punctate appearance to the nuclear chromatin. These two characteristics, when present in a patient's bone marrow cells, make the diagnosis of megaloblastic anemia almost certain.

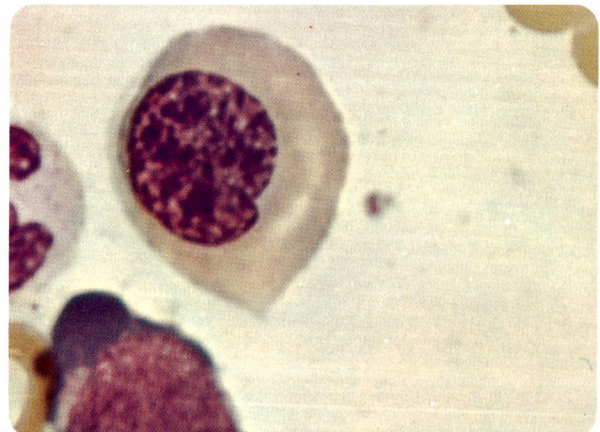

16

Figures 47, 48 Hemolytic anemia

The accelerated breakdown of red cells is referred to as hemolysis. If the hemolysis is severe, then hemolytic anemia will result. In two hemolytic anemias, hereditary spherocytosis and autoimmune hemolytic anemia, small darkly stained cells without pale centers are seen in large numbers. These are called spherocytes. Also seen in hemolytic anemias are cells with bluish gray-staining cytoplasm (polychromatophilia). They represent newly formed cells (reticulocytes) produced in a bone marrow stressed by the accelerated breakdown of red cells. Spherocytosis and polychromatophilia may be seen in any hemolytic anemia.

Figure 47 Spherocytes and polychromasia.

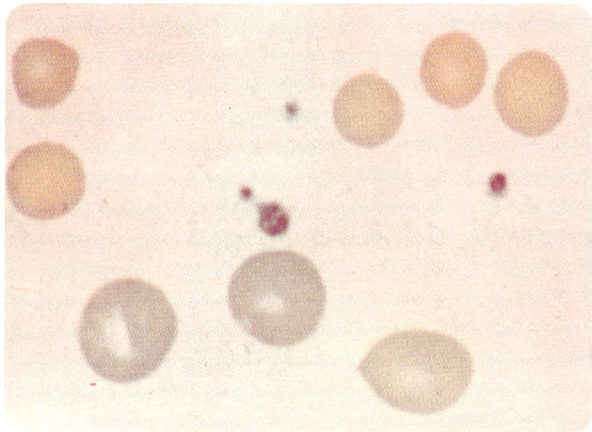

Figure 48
Some other characteristics of hemolytic anemia, ie, the presence of nucleated and stippled red cells.

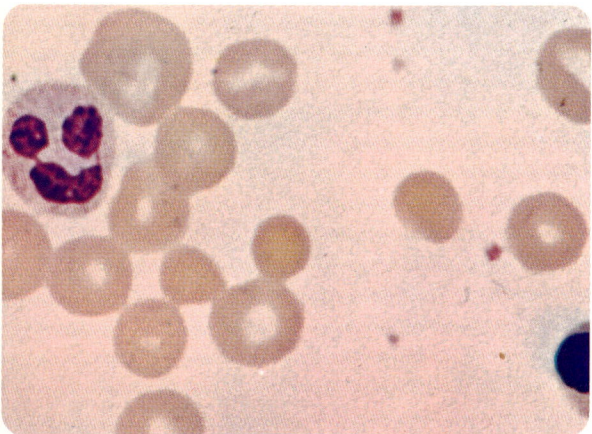

Figures 49, 50 Schistocytosis and helmet cells

Irregularly contracted fragmented red cells, often misshapen, exhibiting marked poikilocytosis, are characteristic of a number of hematological diseases.

Figure 49 Schistocytes and burr cells

Microangiopathic hemolytic anemia, uremia, carcinoma, hemolytic-uremic syndrome, disseminated intravascular coagulation, exposure to toxins, or burns may be associated with formation of these unusually shaped cells.

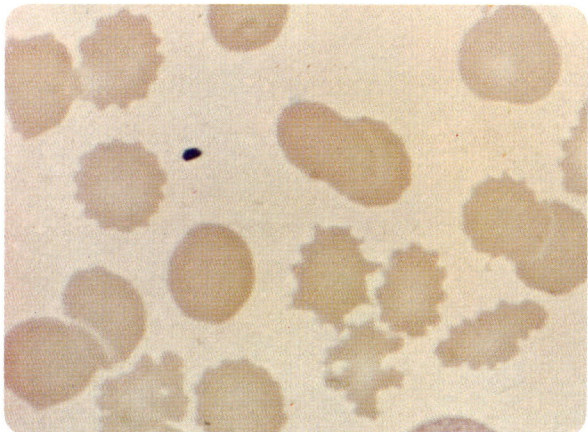

Figure 50 Helmet cells
In some cases schistocytes take on the appearance of military helmets and are, therefore, called "helmet" cells.

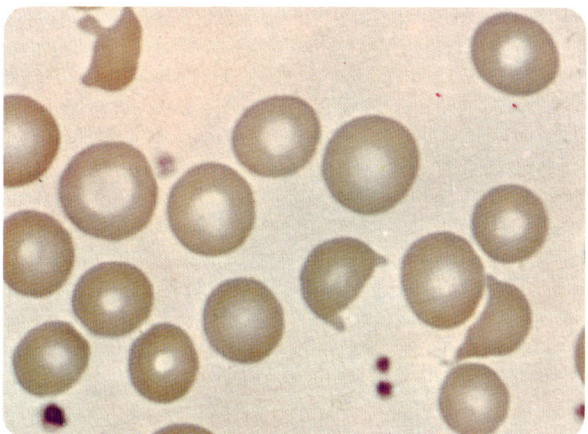

Figure 52 Target cells

These cells have a dark center and periphery with a clear ring in between. They are characteristically seen in iron deficiency, liver disease, thalassemia, and hemoglobinopathies including hemoglobin S and hemoglobin C diseases.

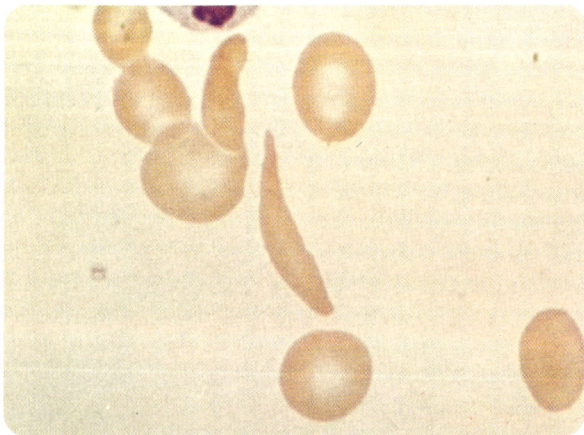

Figure 51 Sickle cell

This crescent-shaped cell is found in the peripheral blood of patients with hemoglobin S disease (sickle cell anemia, S-S) and hemoglobin S-thalassemia disease. When deoxygenated blood from patients having sickle cell trait is examined, sickle cell forms may also be seen.

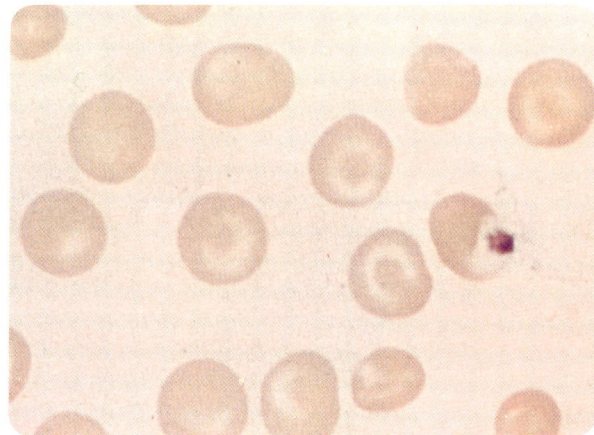

Figure 53 Hereditary elliptocytosis (hereditary ovalocytosis)

Oval-shaped cells are seen in a usually benign hemolytic anemia called hereditary elliptocytosis. In severe iron deficiency, elliptocytosis may also be prominent.

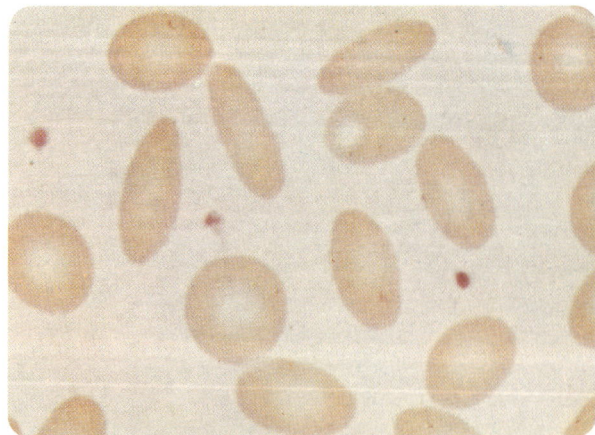

Figure 55

In more severe forms of this anemia there is the appearance of hypochromia, poikilocytosis, and nucleated red cells. Small, round, black inclusions are visible in some cells. These are called Howell-Jolly bodies and are found in thalassemic patients whose spleens have been removed.

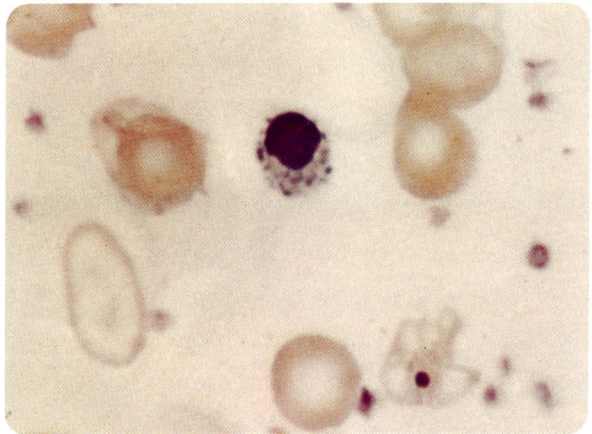

Figures 54, 55, 56   Thalassemia (Mediterranean anemia)
A number of forms of thalassemia are known to exist. In some cases the disease is mild with only minimal anemia and red cell changes, while in other cases marked abnormalities of the red cell are associated with a severe anemia.

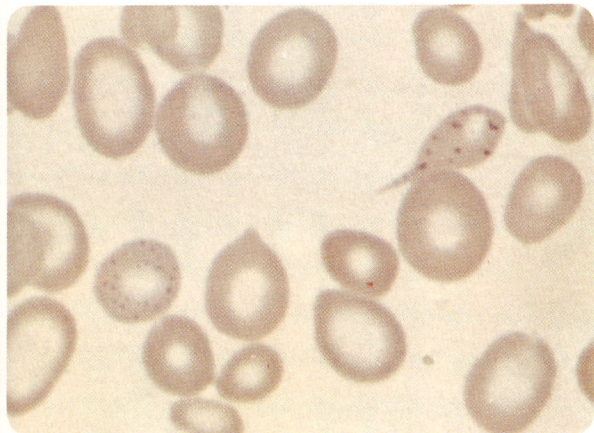

Figure 54
Hypochromia and stippling of red cells may be the only abnormality seen in the mild cases.

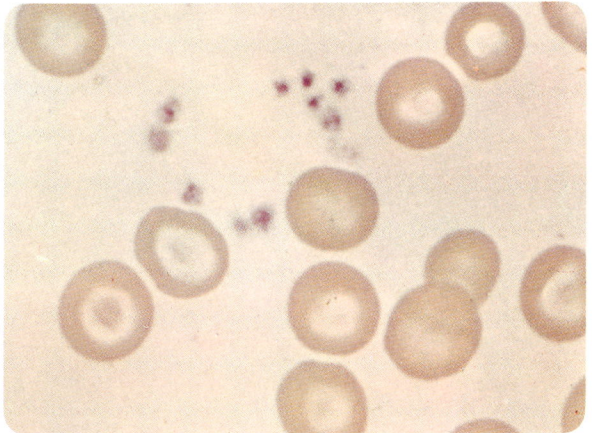

Figure 56
Target cells and microcytes are often present in the thalassemic syndromes.

Figures 57-60   Red cell inclusion bodies

Figure 57   Pappenheimer bodies
These red-cell inclusions are identified only after staining red cells with Prussian blue. With Wright stain they appear similar to Howell-Jolly bodies, but staining with Prussian blue indicates that they contain iron. These siderotic granules are seen in the iron-loading anemias, hyposplenism, and in hemolytic anemias of various etiologies.

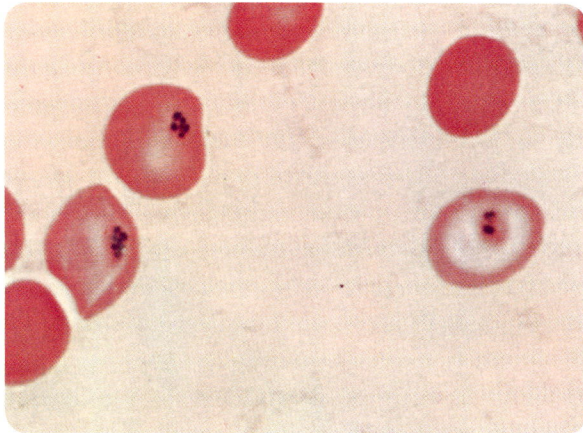

Figure 58   Howell-Jolly bodies
These very small, round, blue inclusion bodies, made up of nuclear debris, are seen in or on red cells. They are most often associated with pernicious anemia or hyposplenism.

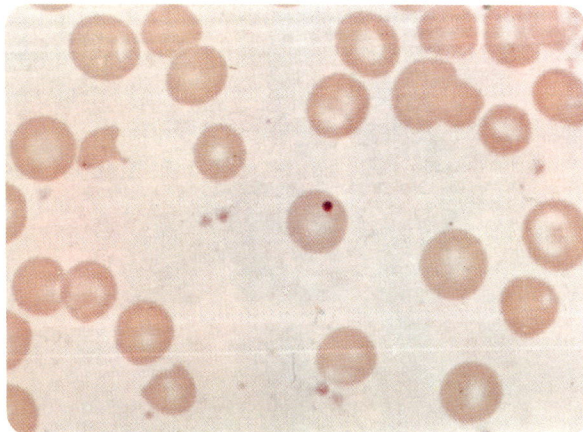

Figure 59   Heinz bodies
These inclusions are seen only after staining with supravital dyes, such as crystal violet. Exposure to an oxidizing drug is often required before they are detected by these stains. They will be seen with phase microscopy but will not normally be present on Wright-stained smears. They are associated with hemolytic anemias due to glucose-6 phosphate dehydrogenase deficiency or to drugs such as phenacetin. Heinz bodies are also associated with thalassemia and other hemoglobinopathies.

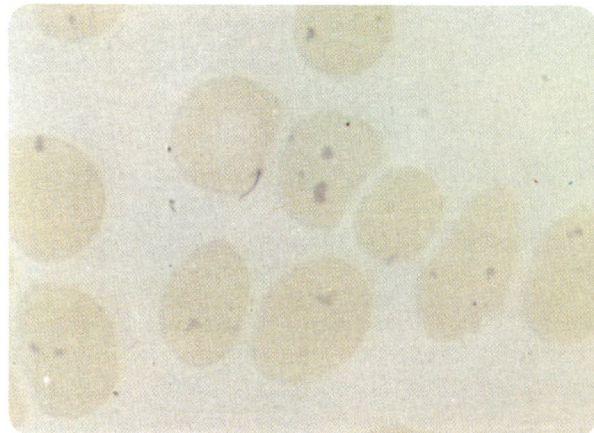

Figure 60   Malaria parasites
Characteristic intraerythrocytic forms are seen in the blood of patients with malaria. These parasites vary in their morphology. Only one example is shown here. They must be distinguished from platelets superimposed upon a red cell.

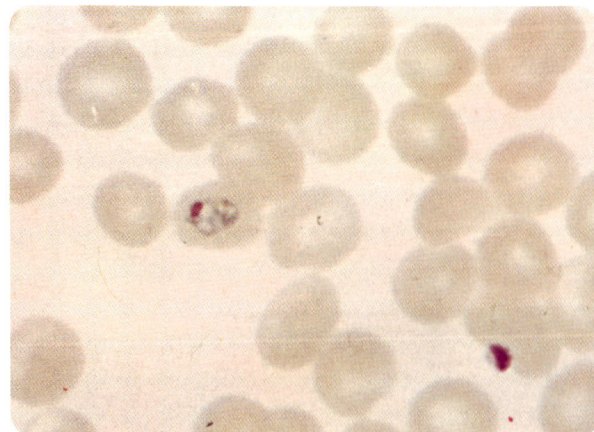